Prostate Cancer:
What Your Doctor Won't Tell You

Prostate Cancer:

What Your Doctor Won't Tell You

Matthew M. Cooney, M.D.

ProstateCancerLetter.com

To order additional copies of this book, contact:
Xlibris Corporation
1-888-795-4274
www.Xlibris.com
Orders@Xlibris.com
108754

Table of Contents

Dedicated to my wife Alana
and our children Seamus, Aidan, Finnbar, Patrick and Katherine.

A special acknowledgement to those who helped me with this book.
These include my father Kevin F. Cooney, Nat and Nancy Cooke,
Ellen Heyman, and the men who gave me feedback
at the Gathering Place.

Learn more about prostate cancer and have your questions answered at
www.prostatecancerletter.com.

Chapter 1

Why your doctor cannot answer of all your questions

1. **Why do you need this book?**

   Advanced prostate cancer is a serious problem and over 30,000 men each year in the United States die from prostate cancer. The treatment of prostate cancer is complex and there is no one treatment that works for everyone. You need to be well informed to make the best treatment decisions that will improve your chances of fighting this disease. This book helps you make informed decisions regarding your therapy.

2. **Do you think my doctor will tell me everything I need to know about prostate cancer?**

   No. Your physician has your best interest in mind but your doctor cannot possibly answer all of your questions. You need to educate yourself about your illness to make the best decisions possible.

3. **Why doesn't my doctor review with me everything I need to know regarding my prostate cancer?**

   There are a lot of reasons why your doctor cannot answer all of your questions. These include: your physician is too busy to spend that much time with you; he may get bored answering the same questions repeatedly; and he might not know all of the answers to your questions. Regardless of how much time your physician spends listening to your questions, you have the responsibility to search for the answers. This book will help you become better informed about prostate cancer.

4. **What do I need to do as a prostate cancer patient to increase my chances of success?**

There are many things you can do to help fight your prostate cancer diagnosis. You need to ask questions, join support groups, read, get second opinions, exercise, and discuss your concerns with your friends and families. You must seek help from others as you take on this prostate cancer journey.

MATTHEW M. COONEY, M.D.

Chapter 2

How hormone therapy will affect you

1. **Are there side effects during my first year of taking hormone injections?**

   Yes. The short term side effects of taking hormone injections include hot flashes and sweats, decreased interest in sex (libido), erectile dysfunction, weight gain, and increase in fatigue. You may also notice decrease in muscle strength and endurance.

2. **Are there additional side effects after the first year of hormone injections?**

   Yes. The longer-term side effects are multiple. These include weight gain, breast enlargement, and loss of some facial and pubic hair. Sexual changes can occur including a decrease in the size of the penis and testicles. Other concerns include elevation of blood pressure, decrease in your endurance, and increased fatigue can be quite noticeable. Finally, issues such as the development of depression and anemia can occur.

3. **How do I maintain my strength and limit weight loss while receiving hormone injections?**

   On average men increase their body fat by 7% while on hormone therapy and lose 3% of their lean muscle mass. It is important that you start and maintain an exercise program during and after you are receiving hormone injections. This activity will help you limit weight gain and preserve your muscle mass while the testosterone is lowered. Setting specific fitness goals and placing the dates and times you are going to exercise on your calendar are essential steps to keep you physically fit.

4. **What are hot flashes?**

Hot flashes are the symptoms of feeling warm, flushed and diffuse sweating followed by chills that occur when the testosterone is lowered from hormone shots or orchiectomy (procedure when your testicles are removed). In the worst scenario the sweating can be so profuse you may need to change your clothes. These symptoms are very similar to what women experience during menopause. The exact mechanism of why this occurs is not completely understood but it occurs when there are changes to the male and female hormones in the body. The occurrence of hot flashes is unpredictable. They can occur once a day or multiple times daily, wax and wane over time, and resolve without warning.

5. **Can medroxyprogesterone acetate limit my hot flashes?**

Probably. Multiple therapies have been tried with varying success. The most effective treatment is medroxyprogesterone acetate. This pill has demonstrated significant decrease in the number and symptoms of hot flashes. The most common side effects of medroxyprogesterone acetate include weight gain, dizziness, headache, and feeling nervous. Medroxyprogesterone acetate can also rarely be associated with an increased risk of blood clots.

6. **Can anti-depressant medications limit my hot flashes as well as medroxyprogesterone acetate?**

No. Anti-depressants, such as venlafaxine, have been compared to medroxyprogesterone acetate for men with hot flashes. Although venlafaxine, which is in a class of drugs called serotonin/norepinephrine uptake inhibitors, can help decrease the side effects of hot flashes they are not as effective as medroxyprogesterone acetate.

7. **Will I have significant fatigue after my orchiectomy or if I am taking hormone injections?**

Yes. The fatigue you may experience from having a low testosterone may actually get worse over time. Generally the fatigue can slowly increase and limit your motivation for physical activity. Over time you may notice significant changes in your endurance and overall strength. You may feel that you are "aging prematurely" while on hormone injections.

8. **Can I limit my fatigue on hormone injections?**

Possibly. Although exercise is important to improve muscle mass, keeping weight off, and lower blood pressure exercise can improve your symptoms of fatigue. Although a variety of herbal remedies and supplements make claims to improve energy and decrease fatigue, these have not been proven in any meaningful studies.

9. **Can I become depressed while taking hormone injections?**

Possibly. The percentage of men who develop depression while on hormone therapy is not known. If you develop depressive symptoms this could occur from a variety of reasons. Depression may occur because of the changes in your hormonal balance, concerns about your sexual function, and distress about side effects such as hot flashes, weight gain, and change in strength. The depression that may develop can vary from minor and transient to severe clinical depression with a risk of suicide.

10. **Can I treat my depression that developed since I have been taking hormone injections?**

Yes. The depression you may be experiencing can be treated by a variety of ways. Talking to your primary care provider, taking medications for depression, and joining a support group, can all help with your symptoms. Do not ignore your symptoms of depression and let it progress. Contact your doctor and develop a plan for the treatment of your depression.

11. **Does lowering the testosterone via hormone injections or orchiectomy affect my concentration?**

Possibly. It is not really known how much, if any, of your ability to concentrate is affected by hormone injections. There are small medical studies that have looked into these issues but are inconclusive. You should still be able to function at your current mental abilities without noticing significant changes in your concentration and memory.

However as we age our mental capacity does diminish and it is unclear if hormone injections worsen our intellectual capacity over time.

12. **Will taking hormone injections or having an orchiectomy decrease my interest in sexual activity?**

Yes. Lowering the testosterone from hormone injections or having an orchiectomy will definitively affect your sexual performance in multiple ways. Before puberty the young man has very little interest in sex and only when puberty starts, when there is an enormous surge of testosterone, do sexual thoughts begin to occur. After using hormone shots, which dramatically lowers the testosterone, your interest in sexual activity will significantly diminish.

13. **Will taking hormone injections or having an orchiectomy cause erectile dysfunction?**

Yes. Almost all men who are receiving hormone injections experience erectile dysfunction. Combined with a decrease interest in sex, changes in the size of the penis and testicles which affect body image, almost all men have a decline in their sexual health while on hormone injections.

14. **Despite these side effects can I still engage in and enjoy sexual activity?**

Yes. Even if you develop erectile dysfunction you are still able to have pleasurable sensation to the penis and testicles. Also even with erectile dysfunction it is still possible to experience an orgasm. Thus men on hormone injections can participate in sexual activity without harm.

15. **Am I at risk for increase in heart attack or stroke because of my hormone injections?**

Perhaps. The lowering of testosterone causes a variety of changes to the body. These include decrease in metabolism, weight gain, hypertension, decrease in muscle mass, increased risk of diabetes, increasing cholesterol, and an increase in fatigue. In total these effects are classified as the "metabolic syndrome" and can increase your risk of heart attack and stroke. The increase in risk of these effects appears to be after one year of lowering the testosterone, although some of the changes can occur in as little as 3 to 6 months.

MATTHEW M. COONEY, M.D.

16. **Will using hormone injections or having an orchiectomy "age" me?**

Yes. The negative side effects of lowering your testosterone will accumulate over time. The weight gain, decrease in muscle strength, thinning of bones (osteoporosis), sexual side effects, anemia, and mood changes get worse the longer your testosterone is lowered. Physical activity and exercise is vital to help limit weight gain, muscle and bone loss, and improve your overall sense of well-being.

17. **If I stop my hormone injections how long does it take for my testosterone to get back to normal?**

Possibly never. The recovery of the testicles to produce testosterone depends on your age and how long you were receiving hormone injections. Younger men, those in their fifties who have been on hormone therapy for relatively shorter period of time (less than a year) will recover normal levels of testosterone generally in 3 to 6 months. However if you are older, had low testosterone prior to receiving hormone injections, or have been on injections longer than a year recovery of normal levels of testosterone could take greater than 9 months. Some men may never recover to normal levels of testosterone even after stopping the injections.

18. **How long will it take after I stop the hormone injections for my body to get back to normal?**

Possibly never. The ability to get "back to normal" depends on how fast the testosterone gets back to normal levels. Once your testosterone returns to normal levels you should notice multiple improvements in how you feel. The hot flashes should stop, your energy level will improve, and your interest in sexual activity should return. Overall these improvements should improve your overall sense of well-being.

19. **Once I stop the hormone injections and my testosterone returns to normal are there side effects that will not go away?**

Yes. Some of the physical changes that may have occurred, such as weight gain, especially around the stomach, loss of muscle mass, erectile dysfunction, and breast enlargement may not resolve.

20. **Can I receive the hormone injections intermittently to limit the side effects?**

Yes. One large study looked at the quality of life and safety comparing men who take the hormones intermittently versus men who take the hormone injections without interruption. The results demonstrated that taking hormone injections intermittently was a safe way to limit the side effects caused by the lowering of your testosterone. You need to discuss with your doctor if intermittent injections are safe for you to limit the side effects based on your cancer.

21. **How long do hormone injections or having an orchiectomy control the cancer?**

This is highly variable. If the hormone injections are started before the cancer has spread outside of the prostate gland then hormone therapy can help control the cancer for an average of approximately 7 years. After these seven years the cancer may become castrate resistant and begin to grow despite a low level of testosterone. If the cancer has already spread outside of the prostate, and then the hormone injections are started, the hormone injections control the cancer on average for about two years.

22. **What are anti-androgens and should I be taking these pills?**

Possibly. The anti-androgen bicalutamide is a once daily tablet that is taken in addition to receiving a hormone injections or having an orchiectomy. This medication works by blocking the signal to receptor for male hormones that increases the prostate cancer growth. Usually bicalutamide is given when the prostate cancer is growing despite taking hormone injections. Thus bicalutamide is given to you in addition to hormone injections when the hormone injections alone are not controlling the cancer. Unfortunately bicalutamide is not very effective. The chance your prostate specific antigen (PSA) will decrease while taking bicalutamide is approximately 20 to 40% and if your PSA declines generally it only stays down for 4 to 6 months.

23. What is ketoconazole and should I be taking this for my prostate cancer?

Ketoconazole is an oral steroid pill that is used to treat fungal infections that involve finger or toe nails. Initial use of ketoconazole in men with these fungal infections experienced side effects of lowering the testosterone, erectile dysfunction, and loss of libido. It was later determined that ketoconazole inhibits the production of male hormones in the body that cause the prostate cancer to grow. Thus ketoconazole has been used to treat men with prostate cancer when the cancer is growing despite being on hormone injections. Ketoconazole can lower the PSA in approximately 20 to 40% of men. The length of benefit of ketoconazole can be quite variable, controlling the cancer for a few months and sometimes for several years. Unfortunately ketoconazole has multiple side effects including dizziness, liver problems, fatigue, and diminished appetite. Also ketoconazole cannot be taken with multiple medications and your medication list needs to be reviewed prior to starting this drug.

24. Should I take female estrogens for my prostate cancer?

Probably not. Female estrogens can lower your testosterone and thus help control the prostate cancer. However estrogens can have a variety of very serious, and sometimes fatal, side effects including an increase in heart attack, stroke, and blood clots. Thus female estrogens are generally not given to men with prostate cancer in light of these side effects.

Chapter 3

Sipuleucel-T uses your immune system to fight the prostate cancer

1. **What is Sipuleucel-T?**

   Sipuleucel-T is a new treatment for advanced prostate cancer. It uses your own activated immune cells to help fight the cancer. It includes the removal of some of your immune cells by a process called leukapheresis (see below). Once these immune cells are removed they are cooled and your blood cells are flown to one of the laboratories owned by the company that makes Sipuleucel-T. In these laboratories, in a process that takes approximately 48 hours, your immune cells are "activated" to recognize a protein that is commonly expressed on prostate cancer cells. Your activated immune cells gain the ability to recognize prostate cancer as being foreign to the body. These activated immune cells are then packaged, cooled, and shipped back via plane to your doctor. These activated immune cells are then infused into you with a procedure similar to receiving a blood transfusion. Once back inside of you these activated immune cells seek out prostate cancer and work with other aspects of the immune system to attack the cancer.

2. **Will I need Sipuleucel-T?**

   Perhaps. Sipuleucel-T is used if your cancer is advanced and has spread outside of your prostate into other areas of the body. It would be an option for you if your prostate cancer cannot be cured by surgery, radiation, or other treatments. Sipuleucel-T is used when the cancer is growing despite your being on hormonal injections that lower testosterone. Usually it is used for men prior to their receiving chemotherapy for their prostate cancer.

3. Are there restrictions on who receives Sipuleucel-T?

Yes. Sipuleucel-T is not for everyone. There is a review process by your insurance carrier to see if you are eligible to receive Sipuleucel-T. You must have advanced prostate cancer that has spread in your body and already be on hormone injections. There must be evidence of the cancer growing while you are on the hormone injections either by an increasing PSA and/or worsening appearance of cancer on CT scans or bone scans. Finally it is recommended for men that are *not* significantly disabled from their cancer. Thus, if you have significant pain or other complications from your prostate cancer Sipuleucel-T is probably not for you. If you have significant symptoms from your cancer the recommendation would generally be to proceed directly to chemotherapy. If you do not meet the above criteria it is unlikely your insurance company will pay for this treatment.

4. How does my immune system work?

It is complicated. Your immune system is measured by the blood test evaluating your white blood cells (WBCs). The immune system has multiple different cells performing multiple different actions. Since a variety of things can attack your body including viruses, bacteria, fungus, and cancer the immune system has adapted over the years to fight these intruders. Multiple different cells, each doing a different task, are needed to combat these varying risks to the body. Thus the immune system is made up of many different cells performing many different functions that work in a coordinated fashion to rid the body of infection or help remove the cancer cells. Sipuleucel-T stimulates the immune system to recognize that a certain prostate cancer protein is harmful. This activated immune system then searches for prostate cancer cells and attempts to rid them from the body.

5. How is Sipuleucel-T given to me?

The first step in receiving Sipuleucel-T is the collection of some of your immune cells using a process called leukaphoresis. You will undergo leukaphoreses not in your doctor's office but rather in another location such as the American Red Cross. Some of your blood is removed using either a large intra-venous needle or a catheter and some of your white blood cells are separated out. This collection of your white blood cells is then cooled and sent to the company that makes Sipeluecel-T for approximately 48 hours. They are then sent back to your doctor's office and infused into you similar to receiving a blood transfusion. This process of removing your blood, stimulating your immune cells, and then re-infusing it into you is repeated for a total of three times separated by 14 days each.

6. Is leukapheresis dangerous?

No. The main side effects of leukaphoreses are the risk of bruising or bleeding at the site of the intravenous needle, small risk of infection, or the temporary lowering of your blood cells including the white blood cells, hemoglobin, and platelets. In general, however, leukaphoreses is a safe procedure.

7. Do I need a special catheter inserted for me to have leukapheresis?

Perhaps. You may be able to have all three of your leukaphoreses without having a large catheter inserted into one of your veins. However, if you have small veins or the nurse has difficulty in finding an adequate vein, you may need a temporary catheter for the leukaphoreses.

8. Does Sipuleucel-T have common side effects?

Yes. The good news is that Sipuleucel-T is a relatively safe treatment for your prostate cancer. The most common side effects are generally mild and include fever, chills, muscle aches, flu—like symptoms, headache, fatigue, and groin pain. These side effects generally occur within two days of receiving Sipuleucel-T and then resolve.

9. Are any of the side effects of Sipuleucel-T dangerous?

Rarely. Significant side effects from Sipuleucel-T are relatively uncommon, occurring less than 7% of the time. The more serious side effects included significant chills, fatigue, back pain, low potassium, and muscle weakness. It is rare for patients to develop a blood stream infection from Sipuleucel-T but this has occurred. Overall Sipuleucel-T is well tolerated and the vast majority of men do well enough to receive all three doses.

10. Can I limit my side effects from Sipuleucel-T?

To limit the side effects of Sipuleucel-T you need to follow the directions of your doctor closely. At the site of your intravenous needle or central catheter, alert your doctor if you develop any redness, swelling, or tenderness. Let your physician know immediately if you develop fevers and chills. Finally if you have any side effects after treatments that are not controlled with rest, acetaminophen, and other simple measures, let your doctor know immediately.

11. Will my prostate specific antigen (PSA) decrease after I receive Sipuleucel-T?

Probably not. The PSA is generally used to assess the response for most treatments with prostate cancer. For example, after starting hormone injections to lower the testosterone, almost all men have a lowering of their PSA to demonstrate the hormone injections are working. However with Sipuleucel-T it is very rare, less than 3% of the time that the PSA will be lowered after the Sipuleucel-T infusion. Although it may be disappointing to not see your PSA decrease after Sipuleucel-T, this does not necessarily mean the treatment is not working.

12. Will my bone scan and CT scans improve after I receive Sipuleucel-T?

Probably not. Similar to not seeing a significant change in your prostate specific antigen (PSA), it is unlikely your bone scan or CT scan will change dramatically (for better or worse) immediately after receiving Sipuleucel-T. Just because your scans do not change does not mean the Sipuleucel-T is not helping fight the cancer.

13. How will I know if Sipuleucel-T is helping me?

It is actually quite difficult to know if Sipuleucel-T is helping fight your cancer. As described above the usual measures of success, such as lowering of the PSA and improvement in your scans, do not usually occur. The theory on how Sipuleucel-T helps is that it takes a period of time to activate your immune system to recognize the prostate cancer and begin to fight it. This time period may occur over months or even years and it not immediately evident by measuring your PSA or reflected on your bone scans. Thus, for men who receive Sipuleucel-T, it is never really known if the treatment is helpful.

14. Will Sipuleucel-T cure my cancer?

No. Although Sipuleucel-T will help some men live longer once they receive this therapy it will not cure your cancer. You will need to think about other treatment options for your cancer in addition to taking Sipuleucel-T.

15. Will Sipuleucel-T make me live longer?

Possibly. Although you will not know if Sipuleucel-T will work for you prior to receiving this therapy, it does seem that a significant portion of men do live longer after receiving this therapy. There was a large trial comparing men who received Sipuleucel-T compared to men who received a placebo. The men who received Sipuleucel-T on average lived 4 months longer (26 months versus 22 months for the men who received a placebo). The probability of surviving three years was also higher for the men who received Sipuleucel-T (32%) as compared to only 23% of the men who received a placebo. Thus taking Sipuleucel-T increases your chances of living longer and also living at least 3 more years as compared to not taking this therapy.

16. Should I continue to take my hormone injections to lower my testosterone during treatment with Sipuleucel-T?

Yes. Your cancer becomes "castrate resistant" when you are taking your hormone injections, your testosterone is lowered, and yet the cancer continues to grow. This is evident by an increase in your prostate specific antigen (PSA) and progression of cancer on you bone or CT scans. You should continue your hormone injections because although the hormone injections are not slowing down all of the cancer in your body they are likely slowing down *some* of the cancer. Once you stop the hormone injections then all of the cancer in your body has a chance to grow and this can cause multiple problems including urinary obstruction, pain and bone fracture.

17. **After Sipuleucel-T, can I receive other treatments including chemotherapy?**

Yes. Since Sipuleucel-T is unlikely to lower your PSA or improve your bone and CT scans you will likely need other therapy for your prostate cancer. Chemotherapy is generally started after Sipuleucel-T if your PSA is increasing and if you are having more symptoms from your cancer. These symptoms may include bone pain, urinary difficulty, weakness, and lack of appetite. There is no minimum amount of time needed prior to starting another therapy after Sipuleucel-T and planning for your next treatment can begin right away.

18. **Can I receive bisphosphonate therapy before, during and after Sipuleucel-T?**

Yes. bisphosphonate therapy is used for men with prostate cancer who have experienced the spread of the cancer into the bones. You are at increased risk because hormone injections weaken the bone strength by causing osteoporosis. Another reason is that by having the prostate cancer grow in the bone this also weakens bone strength. The combination of osteoporosis and the cancer in the bone puts you at increased risk for fracture. Medications called bisphosphonates increase your bone strength and decrease your risk for fracture.

19. **For men with a better immune response to Sipuleucel-T does this mean it is more effective?**

Probably. If your immune system is highly active and recognizes and attacks the prostate cancer this would in theory result in a better outcome in the treatment of your cancer. However the ability to measure exactly what happens to your immune system in your body once you receive the Sipuleucel-T treatment is not completely understood. Preliminary findings suggest that the more activated your immune system is against the prostate cancer the better you will do. All the details on how this happens are not yet fully understood. Currently there is no available blood test that will tell you how your immune system responded to the Sipuleucel-T.

20. **What if I miss my infusion of Sipuleucel-T on the day it is scheduled?**

The sample sent from the company to be given to you is thrown away if you miss your infusion on the day it is scheduled. Since the treatment given to you is essentially your own "activated" blood being infused back into you this must be given to you under a strict time frame. If it is outside of the scheduled time frame, even by one day, the infusion is thrown away and you need to begin the entire process again.

21. **Can I do anything to boost my immune system and help Sipuleucel-T work better?**

Perhaps. Currently there are no specific recommendations to help improve your immune system function and work with Sipuleucel-T to better treat your cancer. However many things can positively help your immune system. These include healthy diet, getting adequate sleep, exercise, reducing stress, and having a positive attitude. There are no proven supplements or natural remedies that have demonstrated a benefit when given with Sipuleucel-T.

22. **Is Sipuleucel-T expensive and who pays for this treatment?**

Yes, Sipuleucel-T is expensive. It costs approximately $31,000 per infusion of the medication. Thus for the recommended three doses it costs upwards of $93,000. However there are other associated costs, including your physician fees, laboratory fees, and CT scan and bone scan costs. Most Medicare and private insurance companies in the United States pay for this medication.

23. **Are there other FDA approved immune therapies available for prostate cancer?**

No. Sipuleucel-T is the only Food and Drug Administration (FDA) approved treatment for prostate cancer that uses your immune system to fight the disease. There are many other supplements and herbal remedies that claim to boost your immune system to help fight cancer but none of these have been rigorously tested by the FDA.

MATTHEW M. COONEY, M.D.

24. Can I receive Sipuleucel-T outside of the United States?

Not currently. The company that makes Sipuleucel-T currently only has enough capacity and logistics for the patients in the United States. The payment details for the medication have not been resolved by other governments outside of the United States. If you want to receive Sipuleucel-T you must be a United States citizen with the appropriate insurance or willing to pay for the treatment.

25. What else is my doctor not telling me about Sipuleucel-T?

Sipuleucel-T is an exciting new medication that is used only when your prostate cancer has spread and it is no longer being controlled by hormone injections. Sipuleucel-T does not decrease your PSA or improve your CT or bone scans. You will never really know if Sipuleucel-T helped fight your cancer. Sipuleucel-T will make some men live longer with their prostate cancer but it will not cure the disease. Ask your doctor if you might be a candidate for Sipuleucel-T.

Chapter 4

Docetaxel and mitoxantrone chemotherapy for prostate cancer

1. **What chemotherapy drugs are used for prostate cancer?**

   There are essentially three drugs that are used as chemotherapy for advanced prostate cancer. They are docetaxel, cabazitaxel, and mitoxantrone. Although sometimes other chemotherapy medications are used for the treatment of prostate cancer only docetaxel, cabazitaxel and mitoxantrone have demonstrated either helping you live longer or decreasing pain related to the prostate cancer.

2. **Can I limit the side effects while on chemotherapy?**

   Yes. The best way to limit the side effects of chemotherapy is to remain as healthy as possibly during your treatments. The risk of side effects is dramatically higher if you are already losing weight, in significant pain, and are already inactive. The least number of side effects occur in the healthiest people at the start of chemotherapy. Those who are significantly debilitated by the cancer at the start of chemotherapy are bound to have more side effects of the treatment. Eating well, getting exercise, and keeping a positive attitude are vitally important in having you limit the side effects that are possible with the chemotherapy.

3. **Do I need docetaxel chemotherapy?**

   Perhaps. You need docetaxel chemotherapy when the cancer has spread outside the prostate, is growing based on your PSA tests or scans, and hormone therapy is no longer controlling the cancer. Docetaxel chemotherapy is a medication given intravenously every 3 weeks. It usually takes about an hour and you go home after the infusion.

4. **Will docetaxel chemotherapy help me?**

Sometimes. You have approximately a 50% chance that docetaxel will help control your cancer. This would include lowering your PSA and possibly improving your CT scans or bone scans. The control of the cancer can range from only a few months to a few years while on chemotherapy.

5. **Will I live longer if I take docetaxel chemotherapy?**

Yes. The average survival time for all of the men who received docetaxel on the clinical trial was approximately 19 months. However how long each individual person survives after taking docetaxel is highly variable. If your cancer responds to docetaxel many men can live longer than 19 months and a significant number longer than 3 years. However if your cancer does not respond at all to the docetaxel chemotherapy the prognosis is worse. Many of these men live less than 19 months.

6. **Is there a limit on how many treatment cycles of docetaxel chemotherapy can I take?**

No. The initial studies of docetaxel limited the number of treatments to 10 but many men today do receive greater than 10 cycles of treatment. You can receive docetaxel without interruption if it continues to control your cancer and you are not having any serious side effects.

7. **Will I have side effects from docetaxel?**

Yes. The side effects you may experience include fatigue, numbness and tingling, nausea and vomiting, and hair loss. Other side effects include the loss of appetite, watery eyes and nose, and swelling of the legs. Finally, change in taste and darkening of your nail beds may also occur.

8. **Will docetaxel lower my blood counts?**

Probably. Docetaxel can cause (or worsen) anemia, lower your white blood cells (which increases the risk of infection), and lower your platelets which put you at a higher risk of bleeding.

9. **Will the side effects of docetaxel resolve or stay with me forever?**

The majority of the side effects of docetaxel will resolve. The fatigue, lack of appetite, hair loss, and return of your blood counts to normal should all occur. If you develop numbness and tingling in your hands and feet this does not always resolve. However this numbness may improve over time.

10. **When should I discontinue docetaxel?**

You should consider stopping docetaxel if your cancer begins to grow while on docetaxel, or you are having side effects on treatment that cannot be alleviated.

11. **Are there other chemotherapy options if docetaxel stops working?**

Yes. In general patients will first receive docetaxel for their advanced prostate cancer and then receive cabazitaxel. If both docetaxel and cabazitaxel stop working to control the cancer, or they caused significant side effects that can no longer be controlled, you need to consider other chemotherapy options. The third option for chemotherapy for prostate cancer is usually mitoxantrone.

12. **What is mitoxantrone and how is it given?**

Mitoxantrone is a chemotherapy given intravenously every 3 to 4 weeks. It works by blocking both DNA and RNA, which are vital to cancer cell growth and replication. After infusion of mitoxantrone the goal is to have the cancer cells die. Unfortunately, like all chemotherapy, it also affects normal healthy cells and this is what causes mitoxantrone's side effects.

13. **Will mitoxantrone allow me to live longer with my prostate cancer?**

No. In two studies it was demonstrated that mitoxantrone can help decrease your pain related to prostate cancer. However, neither study demonstrated that taking mitoxantrone helped the men live longer. The reason to take mitoxantrone is to decrease your pain but not to expect this chemotherapy will make you live longer.

MATTHEW M. COONEY, M.D.

14. **Will mitoxantrone lower my blood counts?**

Yes. In the vast majority of men who receive mitoxantrone you will be at risk of anemia, lowering your immune system function, and the lowering of your platelets which put you at a mild increase risk of bleeding. These changes are temporary and your blood counts will improve once you stop taking mitoxantrone.

15. **Will I have nausea, vomiting and weight loss while taking mitoxantrone?**

Perhaps. About 25% of men will experience nausea, vomiting, or lack of appetite while taking this chemotherapy.

16. **Do I need to worry about my heart function while taking mitoxantrone?**

Yes. Mitoxantrone has been linked to worsening heart function and causing congestive heart failure. This usually can be avoided by not taking mitoxantrone if you have a serious pre-existing heart condition, and monitoring your heart function periodically, while taking mitoxantrone.

17. **Will mitoxantrone affect my energy and sense of well-being?**

Probably. Fatigue experienced on mitoxantrone can be exacerbated with the other side effects of nausea, vomiting, and lack of appetite. In general you should expect to have less energy and motivation for daily activities while taking mitoxantrone.

18. **How do I limit the side effects of mitoxantrone?**

Staying as active and healthy as possible while taking mitoxantrone is important. Trying to eat a balanced diet, getting adequate sleep, and controlling your pain through medications are vital. You cannot limit all the side effects of mitoxantrone. The healthier you are the fewer side effects you should experience.

19. **Are the side effects of mitoxantrone permanent?**

Usually not. The effect on your blood counts, hair loss, fatigue and lack of appetite are usually reversible.

20. How many treatment cycles of mitoxantrone can I receive?

Since there is a risk of multiple doses of mitoxantrone affecting your heart there is a limit on how many cycles you should receive. In general no more that 8 to 9 cycles should be given because of the increased risk after these cycles to develop congestive heart failure.

MATTHEW M. COONEY, M.D.

Chapter 5

Cabazitaxel chemotherapy for prostate cancer

1. What is cabazitaxel chemotherapy?

Cabazitaxel chemotherapy is a name given to a medication that is used to treat cancer. Cabazitaxel is given by an intravenous drip into your blood stream. Cabazitaxel blocks tumor growth and division and thus slows down the growth and spread of your cancer. Cabazitaxel chemotherapy is given intravenously every 3 weeks. It usually takes about an hour and you go home after the infusion.

2. Do I need cabazitaxel chemotherapy?

Perhaps. You need cabazitaxel chemotherapy when the cancer has spread outside the prostate, is growing based on your PSA tests or scans, and hormone therapy is no longer controlling the cancer. Cabazitaxel chemotherapy is generally given after you have been treated with docetaxel chemotherapy.

3. Will cabazitaxel chemotherapy help me?

Sometimes. You have approximately a 40% chance that cabazitaxel will help control your cancer. This would include lowering your PSA, and possibly improving your CT scans or bone scans. The control of the cancer can range from only a few months to a few years while on chemotherapy.

4. Will I live longer if I take cabazitaxel chemotherapy?

Possibly. The average survival time for all of the men who received cabazitaxel on the clinical trial was approximately 15 months. How long each individual person survives after taking cabazitaxel is highly variable. If your cancer responds to cabazitaxel many men can live longer than 15 months. If your cancer does not respond at all to the cabazitaxel chemotherapy the prognosis is worse. Many of these men live less than 15 months.

5. **Is there a limit on how many treatment cycles of cabazitaxel chemotherapy can I take?**

No. The average number of cabazitaxel infusions was 6 documented in a research study. You can receive cabazitaxel indefinitely if it continues to control your cancer and you are not having any serious side effects.

6. **Will I have side effects from cabazitaxel?**

Yes. However it is difficult to predict which, if any, of the side effects you will have from cabazitaxel. The side effects can also accumulate over time. If you do not have a certain side effect during the first cycle of cabazitaxel it does not mean you cannot have that side effect in the future.

7. **Does cabazitaxel chemotherapy cure the cancer?**

No. Cabazitaxel chemotherapy for prostate cancer can lower the PSA, improve your scans, decrease your pain, and may make you live longer but it does not cure your cancer.

8. **Can I still use my other medications if I am receiving cabazitaxel chemotherapy?**

Yes. There are generally very little interactions with most common medications with the chemotherapy drugs. For example, your high blood pressure and cholesterol medication can be taken as prescribed by your doctor while receiving chemotherapy. Always check with your doctor the list of your current medications prior to starting chemotherapy.

9. **Is measuring my PSA important while I am taking cabazitaxel?**

Yes. Regular measurement of your PSA with each dose of cabazitaxel helps you determine if the medication is working. The best scenario is having the PSA continually get lower while receiving chemotherapy. If you have two increases in your PSA while receiving chemotherapy this generally means that the chemotherapy is no longer controlling your cancer and you should move to a different medication.

10. **Will my bone scan change while taking cabazitaxel chemotherapy?**

It depends. In approximately 90% of men whose prostate cancer has spread the cancer goes into the bones. When this happens the bone scan is abnormal and demonstrates different areas where the prostate cancer is located. Generally very little changes occur on the bone scan when the cabazitaxel is working and your PSA is lowered. However if the cancer is growing on cabazitaxel the bone scan can demonstrate new and worsening areas of the prostate cancer spread. The bone scan generally only has significant changes if the cancer is getting worse.

11. **Does my CT scan change while receiving cabazitaxel?**

Sometimes. In only about 10% to 20% of men does the CT scan demonstrate spread of the prostate cancer. If this spread occurs generally the cancer can be seen in enlarged lymph nodes, liver, lungs, or other organs of the body. If the cabazitaxel is helping control the cancer a repeat CT scan, generally done every 2 to 3 cycles, would demonstrate the cancer measured in the body would be decreasing in size. If your cancer is growing, the CT scan would probably demonstrate the areas of cancer getting larger on the CT scan.

12. **Do I need blood tests while on chemotherapy?**

Yes. There are three main blood cells that are checked while you are receiving chemotherapy. These include the white blood cells that make up your immune system, the red blood cells which are the hemoglobin which carry oxygen to give you energy, and the platelets which are cells in the body which keep you from bleeding. All three are checked prior to each treatment with cabazitaxel. These blood cells may be temporarily lowered after each cycle of chemotherapy. Usually this lowering of the blood cells is not dangerous and the blood counts return to normal.

13. **Can some of the side effects of cabazitaxel be serious?**

Yes. There are some serious, even life threatening side effects, that can occur if one or more of these blood cells are lowered. If the white blood cells are lowered significantly this makes your immune system not function properly and you could be at risk for a serious infection. If you develop a fever or signs of infection you need to tell your doctor immediately. If your red blood cells are lowered then you have a decreased ability to carry oxygen in the body where it is needed. This causes fatigue, shortness of breath, and even chest pain for those with heart disease. Rarely are you at risk for your platelets to be significantly lowered. However if this does occur you are at a higher risk of bleeding.

14. Do I have to worry about my liver or kidneys during cabazitaxel chemotherapy?

Usually not. Cabazitaxel is given to you and enters the blood stream. The liver and kidneys help break down the chemotherapy and eliminate the chemotherapy from your body. If you have significant liver and kidney problems either before or during chemotherapy the safest thing to do is stop the chemotherapy until these abnormalities can be corrected. Your doctor will work with you on monitoring your kidney and liver during chemotherapy to ensure they are in good working order and able to function well while receiving cabazitaxel.

15. Can anything be done to limit my risk of infection while on cabazitaxel?

Yes. Using good common sense while receiving chemotherapy will decrease your risk of infection. Frequent hand washing helps decrease spread of germs, avoiding undercooked food or unclean kitchens, and staying away from others who are obviously ill.

16. If I develop a fever while on cabazitaxel what should I do?

Serious infections can occur very quickly while receiving chemotherapy. They occur when your immune system is compromised from the treatment. The most common infections include pneumonia, urinary infections, viral infections, skin infections, and infections that involve the blood. Seek medical attention immediately, day or night, if you develop a fever while on cabazitaxel. Delaying being seen by a doctor if you have an infection puts you at serious risk of harm by not getting the antibiotics started quickly enough.

17. If I develop anemia can I be made to feel better?

Yes. Your doctor can lower the dose of cabazitaxel so that there is less damage to the bone marrow and thus you can produce more red blood cells. A medication called erythropoietin can also be given to stimulate your bone marrow to produce more red blood cells. If your anemia is severe you can receive a blood transfusion to increase your hemoglobin. Although blood transfusions can make you feel significantly better almost immediately the effect only lasts 2 to 3 weeks.

18. Will I develop nausea and vomiting while on chemotherapy?

Possibly. Thankfully the vast majority of men who receive cabazitaxel do not experience significant nausea and vomiting. You have a 20% risk of nausea and vomiting. The nausea and vomiting usually occur in the first 3 to 4 days after chemotherapy and then resolves. Medications are given before you receive cabazitaxe to reduce your risk of nausea and vomiting. You should also ask your doctor for anti-nausea medications you can use at home.

19. Will I become tired while taking cabazitaxel?

Probably. Fatigue can be a major problem while you receive chemotherapy. Approximately 25% of the men receiving cabazitaxel have fatigue although usually not severe. Your lack of energy will occur in the first two weeks after cabazitaxel and then it should improve. At the time of the next chemotherapy treatment the fatigue will recur and this pattern of fatigue followed by a recovery persists until the cabazitaxel is stopped. If the fatigue is severe your doctor may lower the dose of chemotherapy or give you a treatment holiday before resuming chemotherapy to allow your body to recover from the fatigue.

20. Will I have diarrhea while taking cabazitaxel?

Perhaps. You have an approximately 11% risk of diarrhea while on cabazitaxel. If you do experience diarrhea you need to let your physician know. You may need to take medications to stop the diarrhea and help prevent dehydration.

21. Will I lose my hair on chemotherapy?

Sometimes. Hair loss, also called alopecia, can occur in men who receive chemotherapy for prostate cancer. It is very difficult to predict if you will lose your hair from the cabazitaxel. If you are going to experience hair loss generally you will notice some of the hair falling out after the first treatment with a major loss of hair with the second cycle. If you notice clumps of hair falling out consider shaving your head to avoid leaving a trail of hair on your pillow and in the shower. Your hair will re-grow, generally thicker and sometimes wavier as early as 3 to 4 weeks after stopping cabazitaxel. It could take 3 to 4 months to have the hair looking similar to what you had prior to chemotherapy.

22. Can I limit the side effects while on cabazitaxel?

Yes. The best way to limit the side effects of cabazitaxel is to remain as healthy as possibly during your treatments. The risk of side effects is dramatically higher if you are already losing weight, in significant pain, and are already inactive. The least amount of side effects occurs in the healthiest people at the start of chemotherapy. Those who are significantly debilitated by the cancer at the start of cabazitaxel are bound to have more side effects of the treatment. Eating well, getting exercise, and keeping a positive attitude are vitally important in having you limit the side effects that are possible with the chemotherapy.

23. Will the side effects of cabazitaxel resolve or stay with me forever?

The majority of the side effects of cabazitaxel will resolve. The fatigue, lack of appetite, hair loss, and return of your blood counts to normal should all occur. If you develop numbness and tingling in your hands and feet this does not always resolve. However this numbness may improve over time.

24. When should I discontinue cabazitaxel?

You should consider stopping cabazitaxel if your cancer begins to grow while on cabazitaxel, or you are having side effects on treatment that cannot be alleviated.

25. What is my doctor not telling me?

Chemotherapy is used when your cancer has spread outside of the prostate gland and lowering your testosterone, either by hormone injections or the removal of your testicles, is no longer working. Cabazitaxel for prostate cancer can help you live longer, reduce your pain, and improve your overall quality of life. However chemotherapy does not help all men and when it does help cabazitaxel does not control the cancer forever.

Chapter 6

Abiraterone acetate lowers male hormones to treat prostate cancer

1. **What is abiraterone acetate?**

   Abiraterone is a new medication, given as a pill once a day, for the treatment of advanced prostate cancer. The primary treatment of advanced prostate cancer is to lower your testosterone, either by surgical removal of your testicles (orchiectomy) or by receiving a hormone injection. This lowering of your testosterone does control the prostate cancer, usually for several years, until the cancer begins to grow again. Abiraterone is a medication that blocks other male hormones in the body, primarily produced in the adrenal glands, that works in conjunction with your hormone injection. Abiraterone is given when lowering your testosterone by hormone injections has stopped controlling your cancer.

2. **How was abiraterone discovered?**

   For many years it was known that giving a medication called ketoconazole, used to treat nail fungus, had a secondary effect of lowering men's PSA. Ketoconazole lowered the PSA by blocking male hormones produced in the body from the adrenal glands. Therefore ketoconazole was used for many years as an "off label" use to treat advanced prostate cancer. Unfortunately ketoconazole has many bad side effects and cannot be used with multiple other medications. Abiraterone was developed to be very similar to ketoconazole, both in molecular shape and function, but it does not have nearly as many side effects.

3. **If I have had prior treatment with ketoconazole will abiraterone still help me?**

Possibly. Since abiraterone and ketoconazole are very similar structurally there is a concern if you have previously exposed the cancer to ketoconazole that abiraterone may not work. Clinical trials have discovered that if you have had prior ketoconazole the abiraterone generally is not as effective. Also, if abiraterone does lower your PSA it does not work as well compared to men who have never had ketoconazole.

4. **Do I need abiraterone acetate?**

Possibly. You need abiraterone if your prostate cancer has spread outside of the prostate, hormone injections are no longer controlling the cancer, and you have already received chemotherapy. Although abiraterone may be helpful prior to chemotherapy the results from studies examining the use of abiraterone before chemotherapy are not yet available. Thus abiraterone currently is intended for use for men who have already taken chemotherapy and the chemotherapy is no longer working.

5. **Will abiraterone acetate help me?**

Highly likely. The vast majority of men who take abiraterone are helped. This is seen by the lowering of your PSA, the improvement in your bone and CT scans, and the lessening of your prostate cancer symptoms. The more abiraterone lowers your PSA the better effect it will have on you and the longer it will control your cancer. If abiraterone does not lower your PSA, or only lowers it for a short time, then you may be a person that the medication does not help.

6. **Will I live longer if I take abiraterone acetate?**

Highly likely. A recent randomized trial compared over one thousand men with advanced prostate cancer who already had chemotherapy and then received either abiraterone and prednisone or placebo and prednisone. It was found that the men who received abiraterone lived about 15 months versus the 11 months for the men who received the placebo. However this can be highly variable and a significant number of men lived over 2 years while taking abiraterone.

7. **Is there a limit on how long I can take abiraterone acetate?**

No. As long as the abiraterone is lowering your PSA, your bone and CT scans are not getting worse, and you are not having any serious side effects you can continue abiraterone. Some patients have taken abirateone for over 3 years with continued success.

8. **Will I have side effects from abiraterone acetate?**

Yes. The vast majority of side effects with abiraterone are very mild and generally consist of swelling, high potassium, and elevation of blood pressure. Uncommon side effects include liver problems and effects to the heart. Overall abiraterone appears to be very safe.

9. **Does abiraterone acetate cure the cancer?**

No. Abiraterone can lower your PSA, improve your bone scan and CT scans, decrease your pain, and make you live longer. Unfortunately abiraterone does not cure your cancer.

10. **Can I still use my other medications if I am taking abiraterone?**

Yes. There are generally very little interactions with most common medications and abiraterone. For example, your high blood pressure and cholesterol medication can be taken as prescribed by your doctor while receiving abiraterone. Always check with your doctor the list of your current medications prior to starting abiraterone.

11. **Is measuring my PSA important while I am taking abiraterone acetate?**

Yes. Regular measurement of your PSA with abiraterone helps you determine if the medication is working. The best scenario is having the PSA continually getting lower while receiving therapy. If you have two increases in your PSA while receiving abiraterone this generally

MATTHEW M. COONEY, M.D.

means that the medication is no longer controlling your cancer and you should move to a different treatment.

12. Does my CT scan change while receiving abiraterone acetate?

Sometimes. Only about 20% of men with advanced prostate cancer have an abnormal CT scan. If your CT scan is abnormal the most common places the cancer spreads is into your lymph nodes, lungs, or liver. If your cancer has spread into one of these areas this can be seen on the CT scan. If abiraterone is working to fight your cancer and lower your PSA then follow up scans while taking abiraterone can show improvement. The size of the cancer in your body measured by CT scan may decrease over time while taking abiraterone.

13. What is a bone scan "flare" and it is important while I am taking abiraterone?

It depends. In approximately 90% of men whose prostate cancer has spread the cancer goes into the bones. When this happens the bone scan is abnormal and demonstrates different areas where the prostate cancer is located. However, great caution must be used while interpreting bone scan results while on abiraterone because the bone scan may initially look worse. This temporary worsening of the bone scan is called a "flare." Over time, if you are responding well to abiraterone, this flare will improve and the bone scan may actually dramatically improve. The cause of the flare is the healing process of the bone in response to the abiraterone treatment. This healing will quiet down and subsequent bone scans will look better. Thus do not rely on the first few bone scans as you take abiraterone because it may first look worse and then improve over time.

14. Do I need blood tests while taking abiraterone?

Yes. In general abiraterone is very safe but you still need to have blood tests while taking this medication. These include checking your kidney function, potassium, and sodium. Abiraterone can rarely irritate the liver function so liver tests should also be done on a regular basis. In contrast to chemotherapy drugs abiraterone does not frequently affect your immune system or cause anemia so checking your blood counts are less useful.

15. Can some of the side effects of abiraterone be serious?

Yes. Rarely some serious, even life threatening side effects, can occur with abiraterone. Severe headache, cardiac problems, significant shortness of breath, or liver dysfunction could possibly occur. However serious side effects are uncommon with this medication. If you develop symptoms that concern you while on abiraterone contact your doctor immediately.

16. Can anything be done to limit my side effects while on abiraterone?

Yes. The most common side effects of abiraterone, high blood pressure, fluid collection, and elevation of potassium, can be significantly decreased by taking a low dose steroid. By taking prednisone, dexamethasone, or some other steroid you can dramatically reduce the incidence and severity of these side effects.

17. Do I continue to take my hormone injections while on abiraterone?

Yes. Your hormone injections lower the testosterone that is produced in the testicles. Abiraterone blocks other male hormones that are produced in the body. For example, abiraterone blocks male hormones that are produced in the adrenal glands. Adrenal glands are small hormone producing glands that sit on top of the kidneys. Abiraterone works by blocking these male hormones that are produced in the adrenal glands. Thus both medications, the hormone shot and abiraterone, should be given together.

18. Should I be taking chemotherapy at the same time as abiraterone?

No. Abiraterone should not be given while you are taking chemotherapy. Until abiraterone has been studied with chemotherapy it should be avoided and only given with hormone injections.

19. Will I develop nausea and vomiting while taking abiraterone?

Unlikely. Thankfully the vast majority of men who receive abiraterone do not experience significant nausea and vomiting. Unlike chemotherapy abiraterone does not generally cause this but if you do develop nausea ask your physician for medications to limit these symptoms.

20. Will I become tired while taking abiraterone?

Possibly. Fatigue can be a major problem while you are fighting advanced prostate cancer. This fatigue can occur from the hormone injections, anemia, pain, medications, or a combination of everything that is occurring in your body. Although abiraterone may not be the main cause of fatigue, feeling tired is very common from men who have advanced prostate cancer.

21. Will I lose my hair on abiraterone?

No. Although hair loss, also called alopecia, can occur in men who receive chemotherapy for prostate cancer it will not occur with abiraterone.

22. Can I limit the side effects while on abiraterone?

Yes. The best way to limit the side effects of abiraterone is to remain as healthy as possible during your treatments. The risk of side effects is dramatically higher if you are already losing weight, in significant pain, and are already inactive. The fewest number of side effects occurs in the healthiest people at the start of abiraterone. Those who are significantly debilitated by the cancer are bound to have more side effects of the treatment. Eating well, getting exercise, and keeping a positive attitude are vitally important in having you limit the side effects that are possible with the medication.

23. Will the side effects of abiraterone resolve or stay with me forever?

The majority of the side effects of abiraterone will resolve. Once you stop taking the medication the fluid retention, high blood pressure, and the change in potassium levels will improve.

24. When should I discontinue abiraterone?

If your cancer begins to grow while on abiraterone you should consider stopping the medication. You would know if abiraterone is not working by increases in your PSA, worsening pain or other symptoms, or worsening bone or CT scans. If you are having significant side effects from abiraterone that cannot be relieved by a lower dose, you should stop the treatment.

25. What else is my doctor not telling me?

Abiraterone is used when your cancer has spread outside of the prostate gland and lowering your testosterone, by hormone injections or the removal of your testicles, is no longer working. Abiraterone for prostate cancer can help you live longer, reduce your pain, and improve your overall quality of life. However abiraterone does not help all men and does not control the cancer forever. Thus abiraterone can be very helpful in treating your cancer but unfortunately does not cure the disease.

Chapter 7

How your sexual health is affected by prostate cancer treatments

1. **What is "sexual health" and how can it change once I start treatment for my prostate cancer?**

   Sexual health is a combination of many things. Interest in sex (your libido), self-esteem regarding your sexuality, confidence and trust with your partner, all play a role in your intimate relationships. The inability to achieve and maintain and erection, also called erectile dysfunction, can occur before, during or after your prostate cancer treatments. Thus the combination of self-esteem, current status of your intimate relationship, and ability to achieve an erection can all be affected by your prostate cancer.

2. **Will my sexual health be affected by prostate cancer?**

   Highly likely. Regardless of what type of treatment you chose to have for your prostate cancer essentially all treatments carry some risk to your sexual health. It is very important prior to any therapy that you discuss with your doctor what the potential sexual side effects are before you begin treatment.

3. **Will my current health problems put me at higher risk to develop erectile dysfunction?**

   Probably. There are multiple health problems that put you at risk for developing erectile dysfunction. These include diabetes, high blood pressure, cardio-vascular disease, tobacco use, excess alcohol intake, depression, among others. Also many common medications can cause erectile dysfunction such as high blood pressure pills, medications for anxiety and depression, and treatment of cardiac disease.

4. **Can I help minimize my risk of developing erectile dysfunction by controlling my other health problems?**

Yes. There are multiple medical problems that can contribute to erectile dysfunction. These include high blood pressure, vascular disease, tobacco use, alcohol use, depression, diabetes, elevated cholesterol, just to list a few. Keeping these medical conditions under control, such as lowering your blood pressure, quitting smoking, limiting alcohol intake, and keeping a close watch on your blood sugar can all help limit your amount of erectile dysfunction.

5. **Are there medications that I am taking causing my erectile dysfunction?**

Yes. There are numerous medications that you may be taking that can cause erectile dysfunction. These include, but are not limited to, beta-blockers, anti-depressant medications, and other anti-hypertensive medications. Review with your doctor your medication list and determine if there are any medications that you are taking that may be contributing to your erectile dysfunction. See Appendix A for a list of medications that may be causing your erectile dysfunction.

6. **Since I already have some difficulty with erectile dysfunction will the treatment of my cancer make this worse?**

Yes. Essentially all of the therapies for prostate cancer (seed implants, surgery, radiotherapy, or hormonal therapy) can all cause varying risk of causing erectile dysfunction.

7. **If I develop erectile dysfunction after my prostate cancer treatment will this improve over time?**

Possibly. If you develop erectile dysfunction from any treatment method (surgery, radiation, seed implant, or other treatment) the return to normal erectile function may take up to two years to fully improve. However there is no guarantee that you will actually improve

MATTHEW M. COONEY, M.D.

your erectile dysfunction. However, as described below, treatments with medications or devices may substantially help your sexual health.

8. **If I develop erectile dysfunction after my prostate cancer treatment will it affect my quality of life?**

Quite possibly. Previously men who underwent therapy for their prostate cancer developed erectile dysfunction and some of them described a decrease in their quality of life. Concerns about the quality of sexual intimacy, interactions with their partner, and perceptions about their masculinity did occur. In prior studies approximately 50% of men who underwent treatment for their prostate cancer were either moderately or significantly distressed about the decline in their sexual health.

9. **What is "nerve sparing" surgery for my prostate cancer?**

Nerve sparing prostate surgery attempts to not injure the nerves that are essential to achieve and maintain an erection. This type of surgery does improve your chances to maintain potency. However even this nerve sparing approach does not guarantee your ability to obtain an erection after the surgery.

10. **Does the method of surgery, radical prostatectomy, retropubic prostatectomy, laproscopic or robotic, affect my chances to develop erectile dysfunction?**

No. In essence all of the methods of prostatectomy are able to attempt a "nerve-sparing" approach. Minimally invasive surgeries, including laproscopic or robotic approaches, do not diminish your risk of erectile dysfunction as compared to an "open" or radical approach.

11. **Regardless of how my surgery is performed what is my risk of developing erectile dysfunction?**

Even before surgery 40% to 50% of men with prostate cancer already are experiencing some degree of erectile dysfunction prior to surgery. For the men who did not have any erectile dysfunction prior to surgery, the occurrence of developing impotence after surgery is quite high. Reports demonstrate that you have an at least 40%, but even up to a high of 90%, risk of developing erectile dysfunction not sufficient for vaginal penetration after prostate surgery. Be wary of your surgeon quoting you erectile dysfunction rates less of than 50% of their previous patients.

12. Am I at risk for erectile dysfunction after radiotherapy?

Yes. Men usually retain their sexual function immediately after radiation. However as more time passes from the completion of radiation the development of erectile dysfunction may occur. By one year 30% to 60% of men are able to maintain an erection sufficient for intercourse. Thus the development of erectile dysfunction after surgery may not be immediate but after radiation it may develop over several months to years later.

13. Am I at risk for erectile dysfunction if I had surgery and now I need radiotherapy?

Yes. If your prostate cancer is not cured with surgery you may need radiotherapy. Radiotherapy is given if your PSA value does become detectable or if the PSA increases after surgery. The occurrence of erectile dysfunction in men who undergo both surgery and radiotherapy approaches 100%.

14. Is there risk of erectile dysfunction after radioactive seed implant (brachytherapy)?

Yes. The insertion of radioactive seeds, also called brachytherapy, is a method that some men choose to treat their prostate cancer. The cancer is treated by placing multiple small radioactive seeds into the prostate that will kill the prostate cancer cells. The occurrence of erectile dysfunction at 6 months is approximately 15% but this may increase with time. Approximately 25% to 40% of men have developed erectile dysfunction within five years after brachytherapy.

15. What is the risk of erectile dysfunction after cryotherapy (freezing the prostate)?

Cryotherapy is a method of placing small probes throughout the prostate and then running a very cold current through these probes.

MATTHEW M. COONEY, M.D.

Essentially the prostate turns into a ball of ice. All the normal structures of the prostate, including the blood vessels and nerves, are damaged. This damaging of the blood vessels and nerves during cryotherapy and puts you at a greater than 90% risk of developing erectile dysfunction. Cyrotherapy, which can be very effective for the treatment of prostate cancer, has a higher incidence of erectile dysfunction when compared to surgery, radiotherapy, or seed implants.

16. **Of all the methods to cure my prostate cancer (surgery, seeds, radiotherapy, cryotherapy) is any one less of a risk for my sexual health?**

All treatments for your prostate cancer put your sexual health at risk. Although no one method is risk free radioactive seed implants (brachytherapy) appear to have the least risk of causing erectile dysfunction. Approximately 25% to 40% of men have developed erectile dysfunction within five years after brachytherapy. In contrast both radiotherapy and surgery have similar risks for developing erectile dysfunction. The risk for erectile dysfunction from radiotherapy or surgery ranges from 40% to 90%. Cryotherpay has a greater than 90% risk of causing erectile dysfunction and thus put you at greatest risk of developing impotence.

17. **Will I develop erectile dysfunction after hormone therapy or orchiectomy?**

Yes. If you have surgical removal of the testicles (orchiectomy,) or receive hormone injections to lower your testosterone, these will affect your sexual health. In more than 80% of men whose testosterone is lowered from hormone injections their interest in sexual activity, their libido, will substantially decrease. Also the occurrence of erectile dysfunction approaches 100% while on hormone therapy or after an orchiectomy.

18. **Will the use of hormone therapy decrease the size of my penis and testicles?**

Almost always. Lowering the male testosterone, either by hormonal injections or the removal of the testicles (orchiectomy) can affect size. The penis and testicles generally can regress in size in the absence of testosterone to a more pre-puberty state. This may, but not always, improve after stopping the hormonal therapy and allowing the testosterone level to return to normal.

19. Am I at risk for decrease in penis size after having a prostatectomy?

Yes. Although not always discussed prior to surgery there is a very real chance of decrease in penis size after prostatectomy regardless of the type of surgery. Approximately 70% of men will have a decrease in their penis size after surgery and approximately 50% of these will have a decrease in size of 1 centimeter (approximately ½ inch). The average decrease in size is approximately 10% in length and 20% in volume. Nerve sparing surgery appears to limit the decrease in penis size although with any type of surgery this shortening can occur.

20. What causes the decrease in penis size after prostatectomy?

Potential damage can occur during prostate surgery to the blood vessels and nerves that supply the penis. Also damaging to the penis is scar tissue that develops after surgery. The combination of this nerve damage and scarring causes the size of the penis to decrease and these changes are permanent.

21. Do the penis size changes occur immediately or develop over time?

Both. Initially the injury to your nerves can result in the penis "being drawn back into the body." This occurs in the first 3 to 6 months after surgery. After 6 months other changes can occur to decrease penis size. Scarring affects the penis causing it to lose its ability to stretch and limits its ability to enlarge when erect. Thus you can expect both immediate and longer term changes to your penis size.

22. Will sexual activity make my prostate cancer worse?

No. Sexual activity will not make your prostate cancer worse. Physical stimulation and orgasm will not increase the growth or aggressiveness of your cancer.

23. I feel depressed about my prostate cancer treatment. Does this affect my sexual health?

Depression is common in patients who develop cancer. Loss of self-esteem, worry about the future, and embarrassment about physical changes to

MATTHEW M. COONEY, M.D.

your body can all lead to depression. Discussing your concerns with your partner and seeking professional help when needed can improve your depression. Treating your depression with medications may help your mood and ultimately improve your sexual health. You need to be cautious however with some anti-depressant medication because it may cause the erectile dysfunction to get worse. Discuss the benefits and risks regarding your sexual health before you start your anti-depressant medication.

24. **I am experiencing stress in our relationship with my partner. Is this common for men being treated for prostate cancer?**

Yes. It is very common for men undergoing the stress of prostate cancer treatments to develop strain in the relationship with their partner. These concerns can sometimes lead to avoidance of physical intimacy. This stress can exacerbate already existing problems such as financial concerns, work—related issues, family worries, or other matters. Being open with your partner about the changes in your libido, concerns about your physical changes, and self-confidence in your sexual performance will improve your intimacy with your partner. Seeking help from a professional counselor early in your treatment will improve your sexual health and intimacy with your partner.

25. **I currently do not have a partner but I am concerned about trying to initiate a romantic relationship after my prostate cancer treatment. What should I do?**

It is not uncommon for men who have been treated for prostate cancer to have concerns about the changes in their sexual health. This may lead to avoidance of new relationships because of the concern about being embarrassed or the possibility of rejection. Consider being honest with your partner early in your new relationship to discuss your concerns about the changes in your sexual health from the prostate cancer treatments. Professional counseling may help you to adjust to the changes that have occurred since your treatment.

26. **Will sexual activity increase my PSA?**

Possibly. In men over the age of 50 sexual activities can temporarily raise the PSA. After 48 hours of no sexual activity however the PSA should return to baseline. It is not dangerous to you however to have sexual activity with a history of prostate cancer.

27. Will my orgasm be affected by my prostate cancer treatment?

Quite possibly. Approximately 50% of men who underwent either prostatectomy or radiation report problems with their orgasm. A variety of changes can occur which include the inability to climax, decrease in the intensity of the orgasm, pain with orgasm, and leakage of urine during orgasm.

28. Will I have pain with my orgasms after my prostate cancer treatment?

Possibly. After prostatectomy over 10% of men report pain with orgasm. The pain usually occurs in the penis with less often locations including the rectum and abdomen. The cause of the pain associated with orgasm is unknown but is believed to be spasms of the bladder neck and pelvic wall.

29. After my prostate surgery is there medication I can take for the pain associated with orgasm?

Yes. Dutasteride (Tamsulosin) is an oral tablet that can help with pain associated with orgasm. In a study it was found that dustasteride (Tamsulosin) dramatically reduced orgasmic pain in greater than 75% of men and it completely caused the pain to resolve in over 10%.

30. Will I be at risk for having urinary leakage with orgasm after my prostate cancer surgery?

Yes. Urinary leakage during orgasm is called climacturia. This occurs in approximately 20% to 45% of men after surgery. This can develop regardless of the type of surgery that you have (open or robotic). The amount of urinary leakage can vary dramatically from a few drops with orgasm and sometimes significantly more.

31. Can I limit the amount of urinary leakage with orgasm?

Sometimes. This can be a difficult problem to manage. To decrease the amount of urine leaked during orgasm you can limit your fluid intake prior to sexual activity or try empting your bladder prior to sex. Wearing condoms with sexual activity may also help. There is no proven medication that can significantly help urinary leakage during orgasm.

32. Will chemotherapy affect my sexual function?

Probably not. Chemotherapy alone generally does not cause erectile dysfunction. However chemotherapy is used for men whose cancer has spread beyond the prostate and hormone therapy is no longer controlling cancer. Essentially all men on hormone therapy experience erectile dysfunction. Thus those who need chemotherapy because of their advanced disease have already developed erectile dysfunction prior to the chemotherapy.

33. Are there medications and devices that may help me with my erectile dysfunction?

Definitively. The first class of medications that are tried are called phosphodiesterase-5 inhibitors (PDE-5). The current PDE-5 drugs that are available include sildenafil (Viagra,) vardenafil (Levitra), and tadalafil (Cialis). If PDE-5 inhibitors do not help your erectile dysfunction using a vacuum pump is commonly prescribed. If neither of these methods helps the next trial could include medications that are either injected into the penis (intra-cavernous) or inserted into the opening of the penis (intra-urethral) injections. If all other methods are unsatisfactory then surgical placement of a penile prosthesis could be employed.

34. Is there anything I can do to help minimize my risk of developing erectile dysfunction after surgery?

Yes. If you had nerve sparing surgery the goal would be for you to resume as normal erectile function as possible. There is some evidence that taking Sildenafil (Viagra) nightly after a bilateral nerve-sparing prostatectomy may improve the return of spontaneous erections. The taking of sildenafil (Viagra) is thought to improve the blood supply that maintain the erection as well as protect the nerves that enable an erection to occur. Larger studies are needed to determine if indeed sildenafil (Viagra) is truly helpful.

35. **After my prostatectomy will taking medications help with my erectile dysfunction?**

Possibly. All three medications, sildenafil (Viagara), tadalafil (Cialis) and vardenafil (Levitra) have been studied for men after their prostatectomy. Taking any one of these three medications will improve your chances of potency up to 70%. However these medications work best in men with mild erectile dysfunction after surgery and much less well with men with severe erectile dysfunction.

36. **Are there medications I can take after radiation to improve my erectile dysfunction?**

Yes. Both sildenafil citrate (Viagra) and tadalafil (Cialis) have been studied for men who received radiotherapy for their prostate cancer and then developed erectile dysfunction. Approximately 50% of the men who took either tadalafil (Cialis) or sildenafil citrate (Viagra) were able to achieve an erection suitable for vaginal penetration. Further studies to confirm these results are ongoing.

37. **After my brachytherapy, will medications help with my erectile dysfunction?**

Probably. Overall, brachytherapy likely presents the best chance to be able to maintain an adequate erection compared to surgery, radiation, brachytherapy, or cyrotherapy. Approximately 80% of all men who were potent prior to brachytherapy maintained their potency after radiotherapy. If you were in the unlucky 20% who develop erectile dysfunction after brachytherapy sildenafil (Viagra) will improve your chances for potency up to 85%. Thus taking sildenafil (Viagra) after brachytherapy there is an excellent chance you will have adequate erectile function.

38. **Is any one of the three medications best for my erectile dysfunction treatment?**

Probably not. All three medications sildenafil (Viagra), tadalafil (Cialis), and vardenafil (Levitra) may help your erectile dysfunction. However the three medications have never been compared "head to head" to determine which has the best chance to help you. You need to discuss

MATTHEW M. COONEY, M.D.

with your doctor which of the medications may be right for you and possibly even try more than one to determine which works best.

39. **Am I at risk for side effects of sildenafil (Viagra), tadalafil (Cialis), and vardenafil (Levitra)?**

Yes. There are numerous side effects from these medications although thankfully very few are serious in nature. Common side effects include redness, flushing, indigestion, headache, difficulty sleeping, nasal congestion, and visual disturbances. Sudden lowering of the blood pressure and fainting can occur if one of the medications is given with the concurrent use of nitrates or the alpha-blockers terazosin (Hytrin) and doxazosin (Cardura). If you are having side effects from one of the three medications trying another brand may help alleviate some of the toxicities.

40. **If sildenafil (Viagra), tadalafil (Cialis), or vardenafil (Levitra) do not help my erectile dysfunction can I try a vacuum pump?**

Yes. There are several different types of vacuum pumps available for the treatment of erectile dysfunction. The basic principal is that a ring is placed around the base of the penis to keep the blood flow in the penis. Next a cylinder is inserted over the penis and negative pressure is generated either from battery operated suction or manually. This negative pressure pulls blood into the penis. The ring placed around the base of the penis keeps the blood from flowing out of the penis and thus allows you to maintain the erection.

41. **Are there any risks if I use the vacuum pump?**

Few serious. Approximately 70% to 80% of men who use a vacuum device report being satisfied with the results. The risks of the vacuum pump include painful erections and bruising. There is a high drop-off rate with the pump with approximately 50% of all men who start using the vacuum device stop using it over time. The reasons for stopping its use include inconvenience, pain, lack of spontaneity, lack of current partner, or other medical issues.

42. **What types of injections are available for erectile dysfunction?**

There are several different medications used for erectile dysfunction that are injectable. These include papaverine, alprostadil (Caverjet, Edex), and phentolamine. Medications can be injected into the penis (intra-cavernous) or into the opening of the penis (intra-urethral). These medications allow the constriction of vessels which allows the erection to occur.

43. Do these injections work for my erectile dysfunction and what should I expect?

Usually. After prostatectomy the ability to achieve an erection with these intra-cavernous or intra-urethral medications is approximately 50% to 75%. However there is a high dropout rate with their use with over half of the men who try the medications. The main side effects of the injections include pain and scarring of the penis.

44. Can I try a combination of treatments for my erectile dysfunction?

Yes. You may have more success for the treatment of your prostate cancer by combining more than one method of treatment. The combination of sildenafil (Viagra) with a vacuum pump may help you more than either treatment alone. Likewise the combination of a intra-urethral injection with tadalafil (Cialis) may give you better results.

45. What is a penile prosthesis and is it right for the treatment of my erectile dysfunction?

The use of these devices dates back to 1973. The penile prosthesis is usually recommended if all other means do not help. There are several different penile prosthesis devices available. They differ in the number of mechanical parts, flexibility, and whether the pump to inflate the device is located in the abdomen or scrotum. This prosthesis works by pressing a bulb, located in the scrotum or abdomen, which inflates the prosthesis causing an erection. If prior to the penile prosthesis your orgasm and ejaculation was present then this will be continued. However if you were unable to have an orgasm or ejaculation, then the placement of the prosthesis will not restore these.

46. Are there risks to have a penile prosthesis?

Although most men report good satisfaction with the prosthesis there are some potential serious complications. These include risk of infection, skin injury and erosion, pain, and possibility of accidental inflation during exercise. The prosthesis can be removed by your urologist if there are any complications or you do not want to have it anymore.

47. **My prostate cancer is cured but I have a low testosterone level causing erectile dysfunction. If I take testosterone replacement will this cause my cancer to recur?**

Probably not. As you get older you may develop a lower testosterone level which is a normal function of aging. One side effect of having low testosterone is erectile dysfunction. If you have had a curative treatment for your prostate cancer, such as surgery or radiation, and there is no evidence that the cancer has recurred, then giving you testosterone replacement will not make the cancer return. Giving you testosterone does not cause the cancer. However if you still have prostate cancer in your body giving testosterone replacement may cause your PSA to increase and possibly even the cancer to spread. Therefore many physicians are reluctant to give you testosterone replacement after your prostate cancer treatment if it is not yet known for sure that your cancer is cured.

48. **Is it ever safe to take testosterone replacement if I had a history of prostate cancer?**

Sometimes. It is safe to take testosterone replacement if you have been cured of your prostate cancer. Waiting at least 5 years without any evidence of the prostate cancer from recurring would be advisable prior to starting testosterone replacement.

49. **Can I still enjoy sexual activity if I have erectile dysfunction from my prostate cancer treatments?**

Yes. If you have developed erectile dysfunction and intercourse is not possible it does not mean your sex life is over. You can express your intimacy through use of your hands, mouths, tongues and lips. Sensual massage, adult toys, and other means can replace the intercourse and reestablish intimacy with your partner.

50. What is my doctor not telling me?

Your sexual health is the combination of desire, intimacy with your partner, and physical contact. Your libido, the desire for sexual contact, can be affected by prostate cancer treatments that lower the testosterone. Also your intimacy with your partner may be affected by a change in your body image or self-confidence. Finally erectile dysfunction, the inability to achieve and maintain an erection, may occur after your treatment. You need to discuss with your doctor the effects of any and all of your treatments on your libido, intimacy, and erectile function prior to initiating any treatments. This will allow you and your partner to prepare for changes in your sexual health during the treatment of your prostate cancer and seek treatment when possible.

Chapter 8

Why exercise is important for your prostate cancer treatments

1. **Are there health benefits to keep physically fit during prostate cancer treatments?**

   Absolutely. The benefits of starting and maintaining an exercise program since you have prostate cancer are many. Benefits include increase in muscle strength, improved energy, a decrease in stress levels, lowering of anxiety, improved sleep, weight control, and an improvement in the overall sense of well-being. Exercise can also lower your risk factors for cardiovascular disease.

2. **Why doesn't my cancer doctor talk to me about exercise?**

   Unfortunately most of the doctors who care for patients with prostate cancer talk very little about the importance of exercising with their patients. Many physicians have very limited knowledge about exercise programs and do not know enough to make any specific recommendations. Also your doctor may not exercise and feels self-conscious telling you to get in shape. However just because your doctor does not talk about exercise does not mean it is not important for you. Exercise is a vital component for your health and well-being as you fight prostate cancer.

3. **Do I need to see my doctor first prior to starting an exercise program?**

   Yes. Everyone has a different level of fitness based on their age, other medical conditions, prior levels of activity, and access to exercise programs. Your stage of disease, treatments planned, and risk of problems from your prostate cancer make your exercise needs unique. Do not start an exercise regimen first without talking to a doctor to help determine which program is right for you.

4. **Should I work with an exercise specialist, sports trainer, physical therapist, or other professional during my exercise program?**

Whenever possible. Once your doctor has allowed you to start an exercise program working with a trained professional to help set up a fitness program is an excellent idea. This professional can gauge your current fitness status, review your areas that need improvement, and help set goals for you to achieve. This professional can also work with you to show you the correct technique on specific exercises so that you do not injure yourself. Finally, a good fitness trainer provides encouragement and motivation for you to continue your exercise schedule.

5. **Are there common barriers to starting an exercise program if you have prostate cancer?**

Yes, although in essence all of these barriers are ultimately just excuses. The most common reasons men give to not exercising include being "too busy" and having "no will power." Neither of these reasons is good enough to keep you from improving your health and well-being by starting a fitness program. We will discuss strategies on how you can start a program, maintain and improve your fitness, and keep you motivated to exercise even on days when you do not want to.

6. **I have urinary incontinence from my prostate cancer treatments, will exercise make this worse?**

Incontinence can occur after surgery, radiation therapy, or brachytherapy (seed implants). Although exercise will not make the incontinence worse many men feel reluctant to get active if they are leaking a lot of urine. The recommendation is even if you have urinary incontinence you still need to begin an exercise program. By wearing absorbent pads you can still exercise even if you have incontinence.

7. **Does it matter if I start my exercise program during treatment or after treatment?**

Yes and no. The recommendation is to start an exercise program as soon as you start your prostate cancer treatments (once you have been approved by your physician). Studies have shown that men benefit both from exercising during their cancer treatments as well as from continuing exercise programs long after their cancer treatments are completed. It is never too late to begin a fitness program. Set goals now and begin to improve your life by exercising.

8. **I have completed my surgery (or radiation) should I consider a fitness program?**

Yes. After dealing with cancer it is a good time to change your life for the better which includes an exercise program. Although most men who underwent surgery or radiation are cured although there is no guarantee that your cancer will not return. If the cancer does recur, you will be much more physically fit to undertake the needed treatments or medications that will be used to battle your prostate cancer by starting an exercise program now.

9. **How many times a week and for how long do I need to exercise to gain benefit from the program?**

The more times you exercise the better. Reasonable goals include exercising three times a week for at least 30 minutes each time. Programs that combine both exercises such as walking, running, biking or swimming with resistance training may be of most benefit. Your goals, including increasing your aerobic capacity with improving your muscle and bone strength, will keep you fit as possible.

10. **Is there one exercise or training program more beneficial than others for my prostate cancer treatments?**

No. A variety of exercise programs have been evaluated for patients with cancer. These include, but are not limited to, walking, resistance training, weight training, running, among others. All appear to have benefit for your treatments and well-being. Your exercise program needs to be specific for your needs based on current medical conditions and limitations. The best advice is to pick an exercise regimen that your doctor thinks is safe for you and that you enjoy doing. If you do not enjoy the activity it is unlikely you will continue the exercise regimen in the long term.

11. Will group exercise be a good option for me?

Yes. The best studies that demonstrated the biggest benefit of exercise all had men exercising as a group. Nothing motivates you more than knowing others are counting on you to show up for your work out. This team approach to getting healthy, working out with others, will help motivate you even on the days you really do not want to sweat.

12. Will strength training help me?

Yes. Strength training is isolating muscles, or muscle groups, and stressing these by using resistance exercises. Examples include using weights, resistance bands, and machines that give resistance to the movement to stress the muscle. Strength training will improve muscle mass and increase bone strength.

13. What if I am too busy to exercise?

The reality is you are not too busy to exercise. You must put your work out on the calendar and stick to the time and place of the appointment. Your time to exercise should be protected on your calendar and is just as important as any other activity or meeting. If you do not take care of yourself and exercise no one else will.

14. How will I know if my exercise program has any benefit for me?

You must keep a log of all your work outs and what you accomplished. Record how far you walked, ran, swam or other activity. Record each set of resistance training and write these down. Review what you did this month and compare to last month's work outs. Finally writing down specific exercise goals where you can read them before each work out helps motivate you to keep going even at the times you want to take a day off.

15. Will staying physically fit help lessen my erectile dysfunction?

Perhaps. Erectile dysfunction can occur from a variety of causes including low testosterone, damage from your surgery or radiation, diabetes, high blood pressure, high cholesterol, and other risk factors. Exercise improves your cardiovascular fitness by increasing blood flow

MATTHEW M. COONEY, M.D.

to all parts of the body, including the penis. Although exercise alone will not fix erectile dysfunction it may help your overall fitness which will limit the progression of your erectile dysfunction.

16. **Will hormone therapy, even if used only for a short time, affect my level of fitness?**

Absolutely. Hormone therapy for prostate cancer lowers your testosterone. With a lower testosterone multiple side effects occur including increased fatigue, loss of muscle mass, and the development of the thinning of bones (osteopenia). It has been demonstrated that exercising on a regular basis while receiving hormone therapy for prostate cancer can improve muscle mass, reduce fatigue, and improve the overall sense of well-being.

17. **Will my cardiovascular shape be affected by hormone therapy?**

Yes. Your cardiovascular fitness is defined as your ability to perform exercise such as walking, running, and swimming. Your cardiovascular fitness will be impacted by hormone therapy several ways. The first is by the increased fatigue you will experience by having a lowered testosterone. You will be at increased risk of gaining weight which will make aerobic exercise more difficult. Finally by being more fatigued and gaining weight this will put you at risk for an increase in your blood pressure which may cause your heart to work harder during exercise. Staying physically fit you can limit all of these side effects to a minimum.

18. **Will hormone therapy affect my muscle strength?**

Absolutely. Men on average can lose up to 5% of their muscle mass and decrease their muscle strength up to 25% on hormone therapy. Your level of physical fitness will decrease to a performance of someone 10 to 20 years older.

19. **Will hormone therapy affect my bone strength?**

Yes. The thinning of your bones on hormone therapy, called osteopenia, will occur while on hormone therapy. You will also be at a four times increase risk of falling and fracture on hormonal therapy.

20. **On hormone therapy will I get fat?**

Quite possibly. With the lowering of your testosterone and slowing of your metabolism you are at great risk of gaining weight. Men can gain on average 10% to 20% increase in fat weight which could easily mean gaining 20 to 40 extra pounds. Exercise and a healthy diet are vital to combat this weight gain.

21. **Can exercise help with my muscles mass, bone health, and limit weight gain?**

Yes. Multiple studies demonstrate that exercise increases your muscle strength. Some studies have demonstrated over a 100% increase in muscle strength with regular resistance exercises. The improvement of bone density, which decreases your fracture risk, also occurs with a fitness program. Finally weight gain can be minimized with a regular exercise.

22. **How do I know if I have cancer related fatigue?**

Cancer related fatigue is a persistent sense of physical, emotional, and or cognitive exhaustion out of proportion to daily activity related to your having cancer or your cancer treatments. Your fatigue related to prostate cancer can be from a variety of reasons including low testosterone, sleep disturbances, stress, anemia, depression, medications, and chemotherapy, among others. You need to be evaluated by your physician to help determine what factors are contributing to your fatigue.

23. **Can exercise help limit my fatigue, sense of well-being, and help decrease anxiety?**

Yes. Multiple studies have demonstrated that exercising decreases fatigue and improve overall quality of life. Your fitness program will help you decrease your stress and lower levels of anxiety.

24. **Will I lose a lot of weight and change my body dramatically with an exercise program?**

Probably not. Exercise will help you increase your strength, build stamina, and control your weight. However it is not common to lose a huge amount of weight and dramatically change your appearance. Do not be discouraged if you do not look different in the mirror. It is more important than you are exercising on a regular basis which has multiple beneficial effects on your health.

25. **What is my doctor not telling me?**

Your doctor does not have enough time to stress the importance of exercise as you battle prostate cancer. Exercise regimens will keep you fit and improve your energy level, muscle strength, and overall sense of well-being. You need to find a fitness professional to help design a regimen that will keep you healthy as you receive your prostate cancer treatments. Keep exercising at least 3 times a week and keep a record of your progress.

Appendix A.

List of medication that may cause erectile dysfunction.

Amlodipine
Atomoxetine
Atorvastatin
Carvedilol
Degarelix
Desvenlafaxine
Duloxetine
Fluoxetine
Fluvastatin
Goserelin
Hydrochlorothiazide
Methyphenidate
Olanzapine
Pravastatin
Risperidone
Rosuvastatin
Simvastatin
Telmisartan
Terbinafine
Trazadone
Triptorelin
Vigabatrin

www.ingramcontent.com/pod-product-compliance
Lightning Source LLC
Chambersburg PA
CBHW021252280526
45784CB00005B/2342